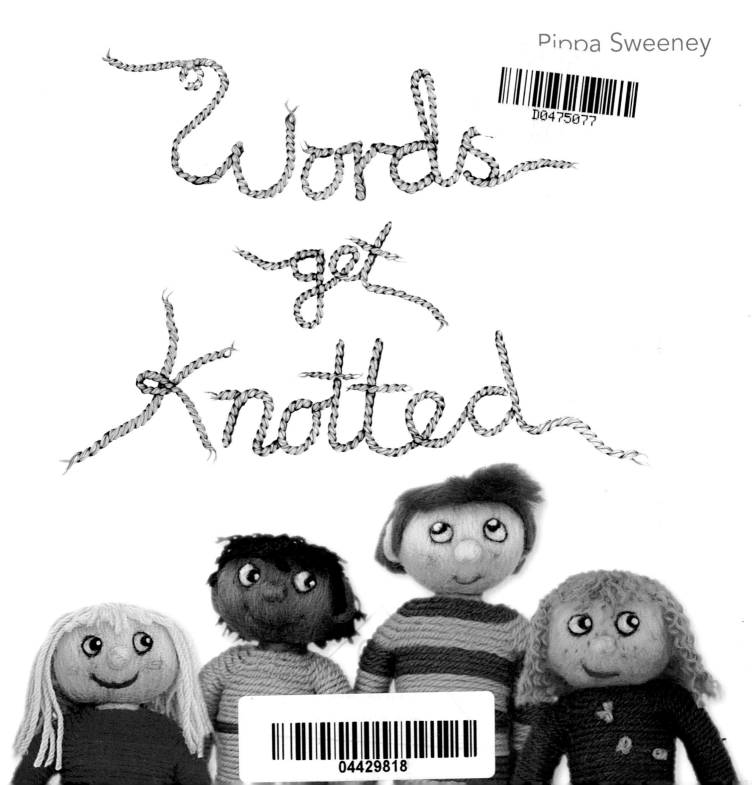

Pippa Sweeney

Words get Knotted

Published 2012 by Featherstone Education
Bloomsbury Publishing plc
50 Bedford Square, London,
www.acblack.com

ISBN HB 978-1-4081-7589-7
      PB 978-1-4081-8188-1

Text and illustration © Pippa Sweeney 2012
Photographs by Beatrlce Forshall

Dedicated to Mike, Rebecca, Calum and Freya with love

Printed in China by C&C Offset Printing Co Ltd, Shenzhen, Guangdong

This book is produced using paper that is made from wood grown in
managed, sustainable forests. It is natural, renewable and recyclable.
The logging and manufacturing processes conform to the environmental
regulations of the country of origin.

To see our full range of titles visit www.acblack.com

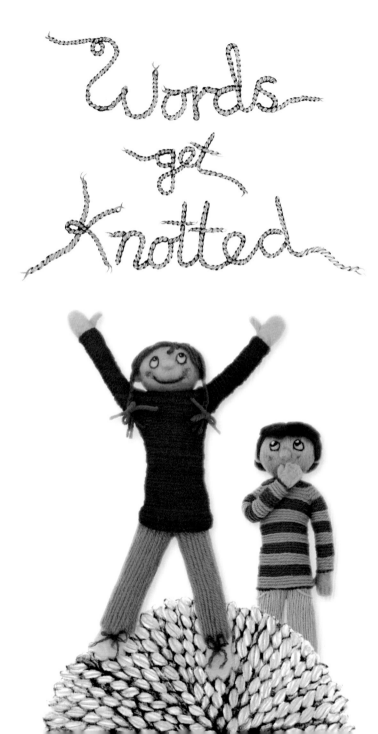

Some people find words easy...

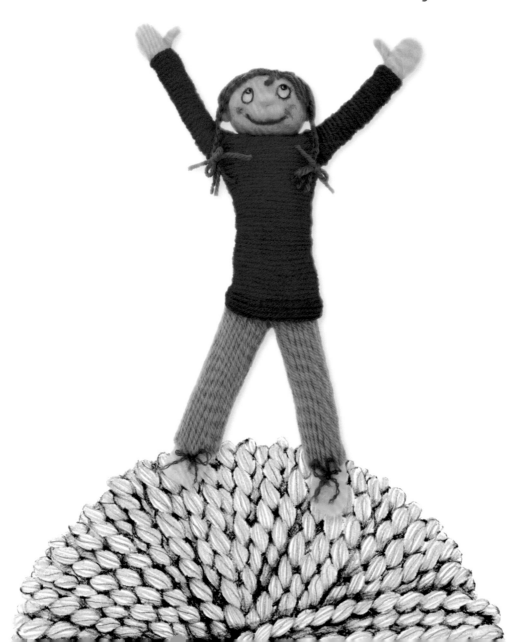

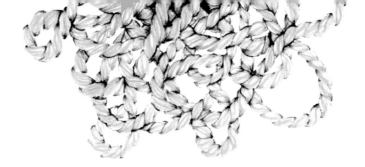

while others find them tricky.

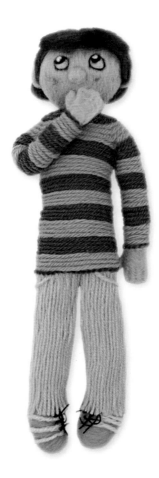

Some people say...

words and
writing
are like ...

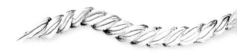

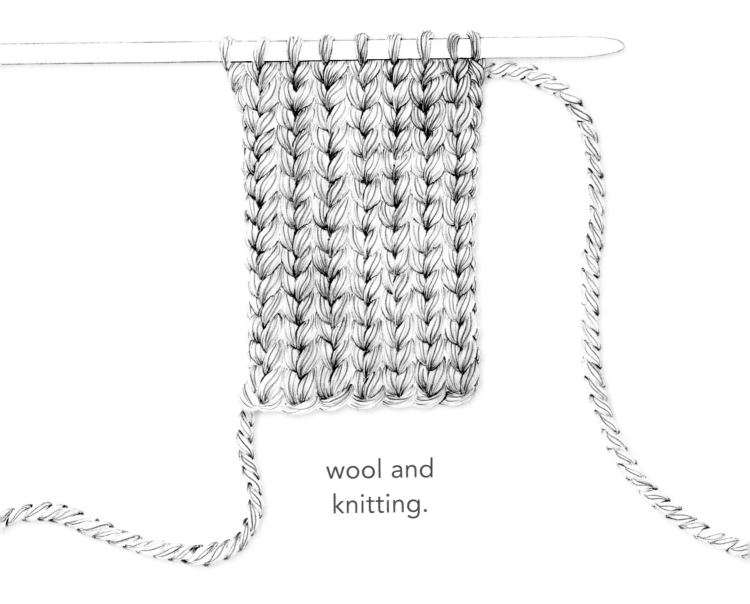

wool and
knitting.

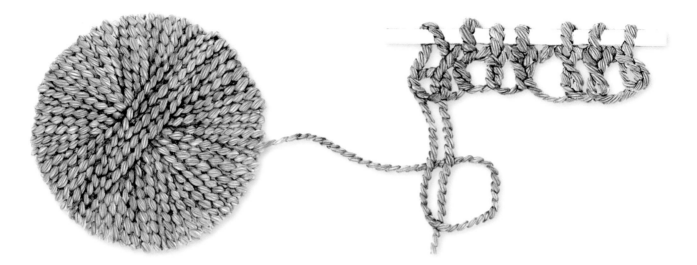

You have to decide
which words to use.

Starting may take
a little time...

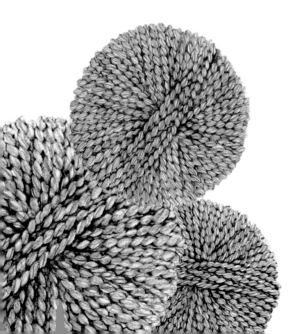

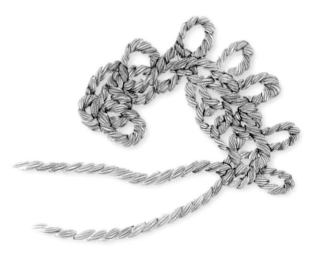

and you may
make mistakes.

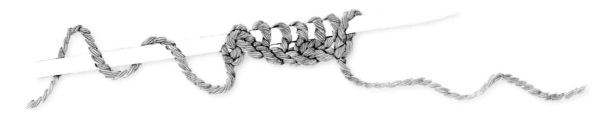

But if you start again,
and don't worry if you...

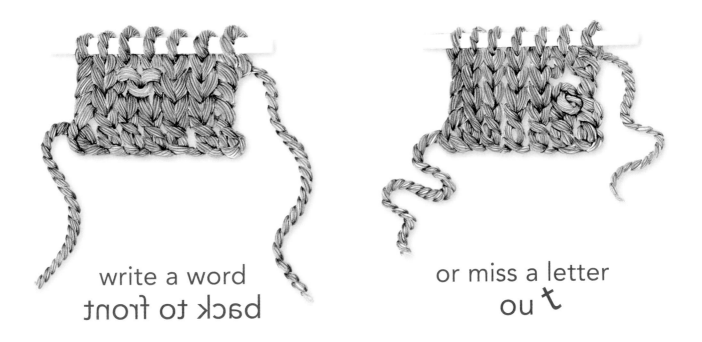

write a word
back to front

or miss a letter
ou t

or if you write something

differntly each time

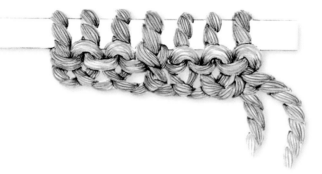

diferently each time

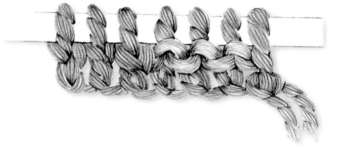

differently each time

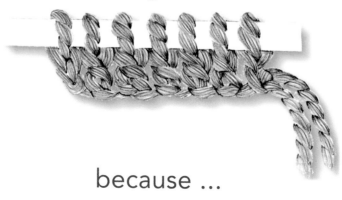

because ...

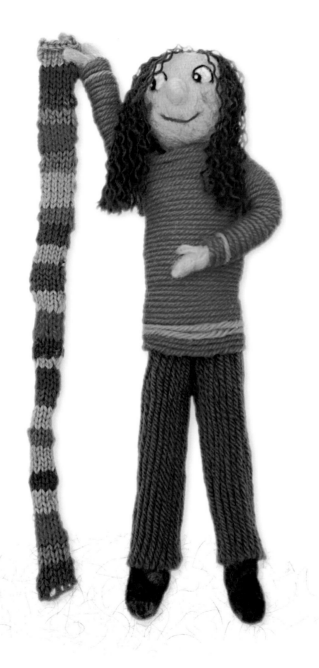

you can do it!

If people find reading and writing tricky, other things may be difficult too.

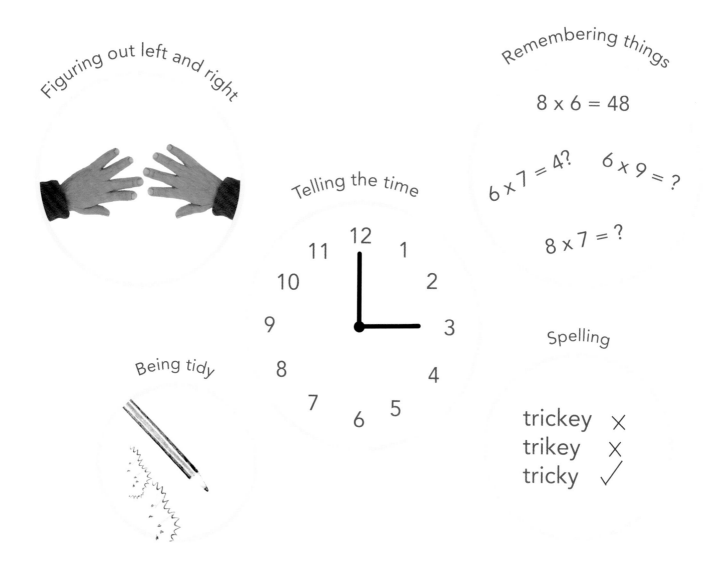

Figuring out left and right

Remembering things

$8 \times 6 = 48$

$6 \times 7 = 4?$ $6 \times 9 = ?$

$8 \times 7 = ?$

Telling the time

Being tidy

Spelling

trickey ✗
trikey ✗
tricky ✓

This is because their brains work in a different way, not because they are less clever.

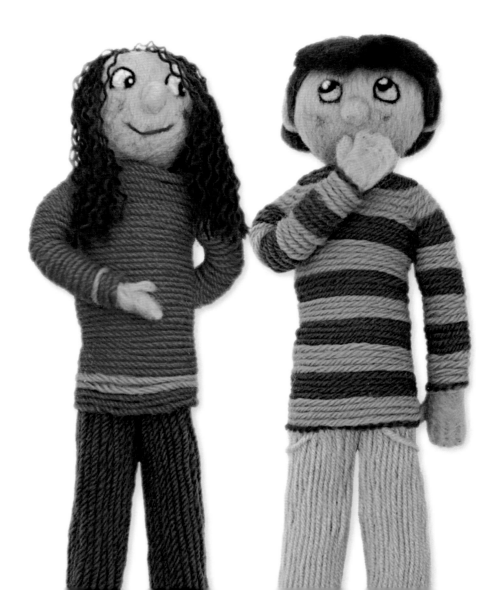

Copying from the board may be slow...

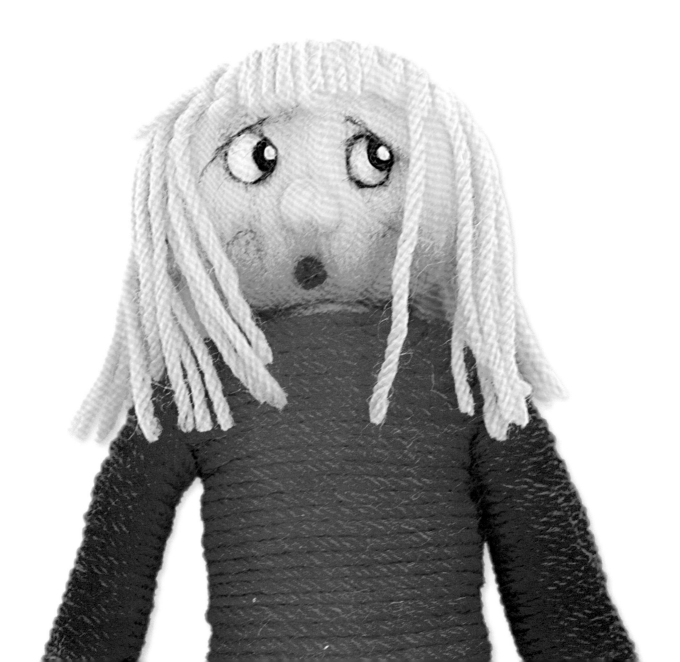

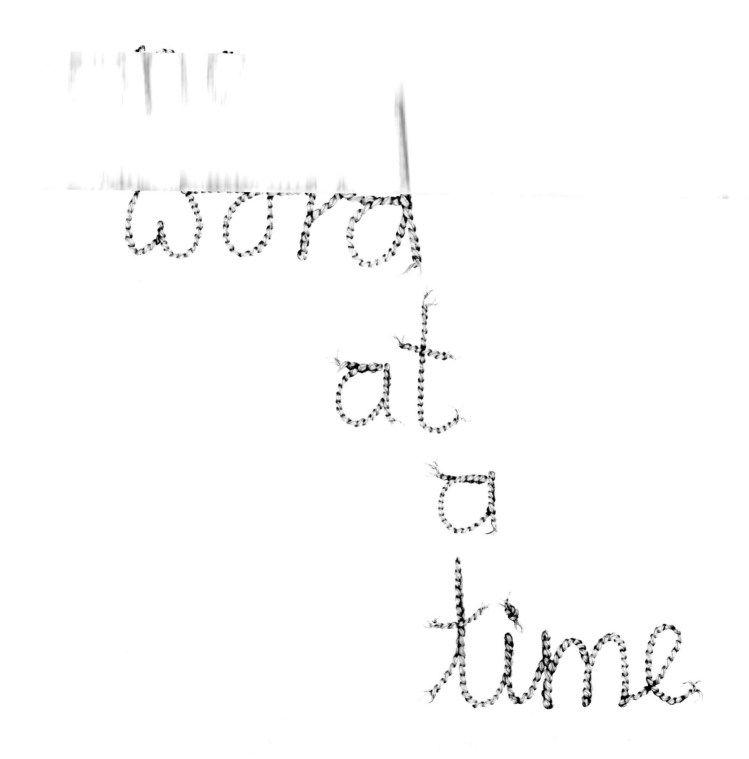

word at a time

or they may have a great idea for a story...

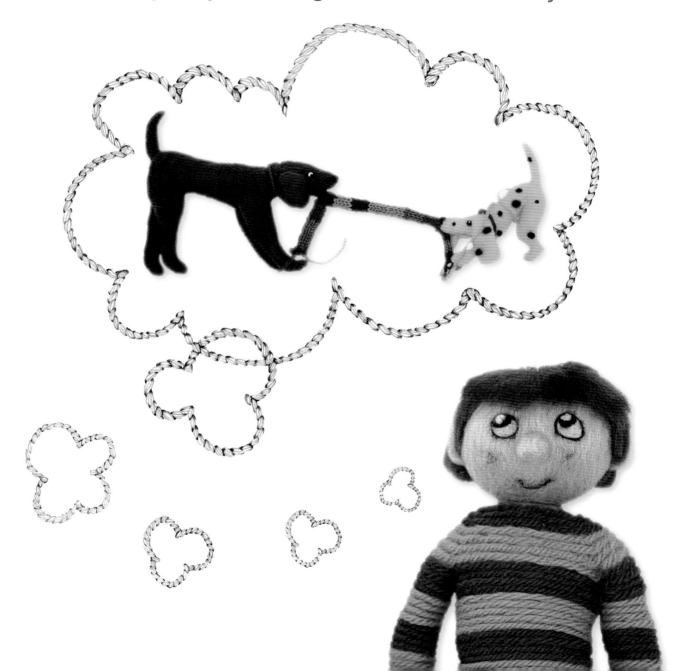

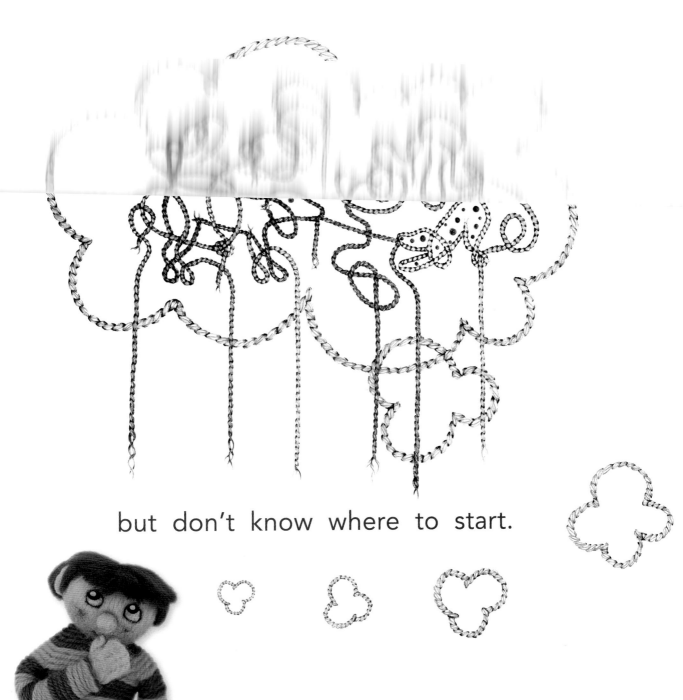

but don't know where to start.

Sometimes people have to work hard at their reading and when they read aloud they may have a...

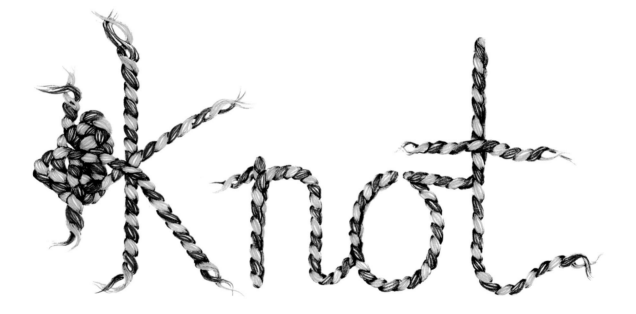

in their tummy.

They may have to read something...

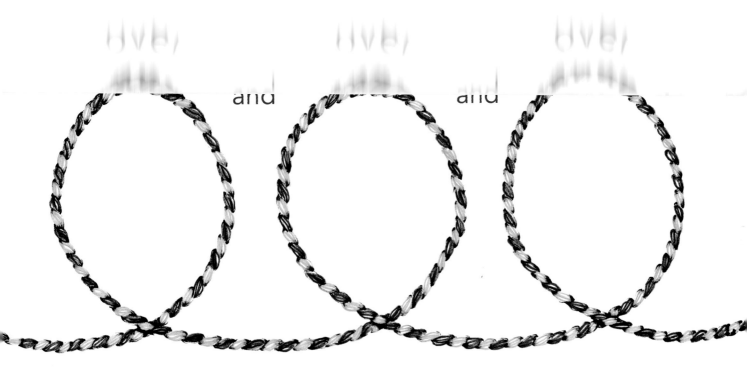

until it makes sense.

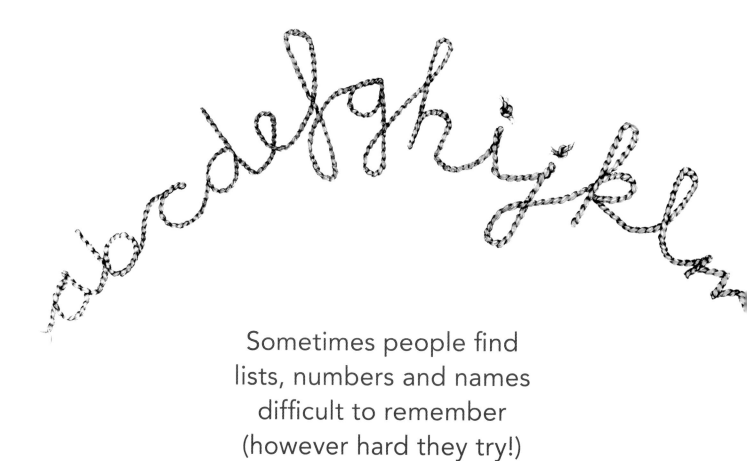

Sometimes people find
lists, numbers and names
difficult to remember
(however hard they try!)

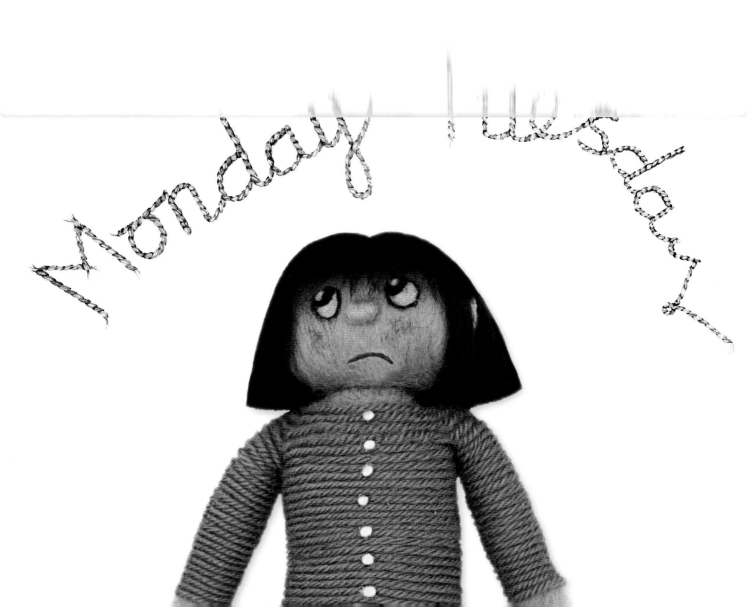

If they find words tricky, someone else in their family may too. Perhaps, when they want to say something...

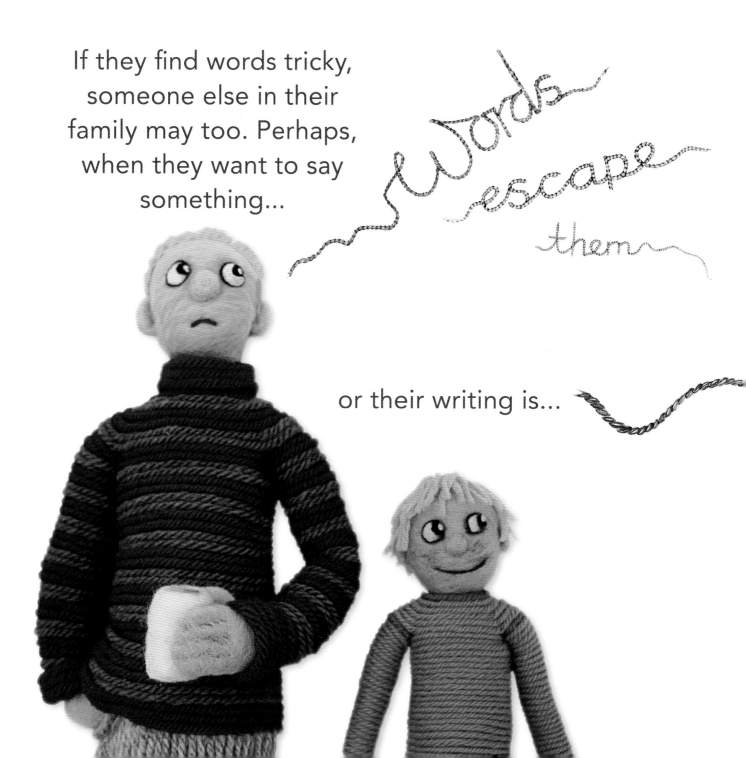

Words escape them

or their writing is...

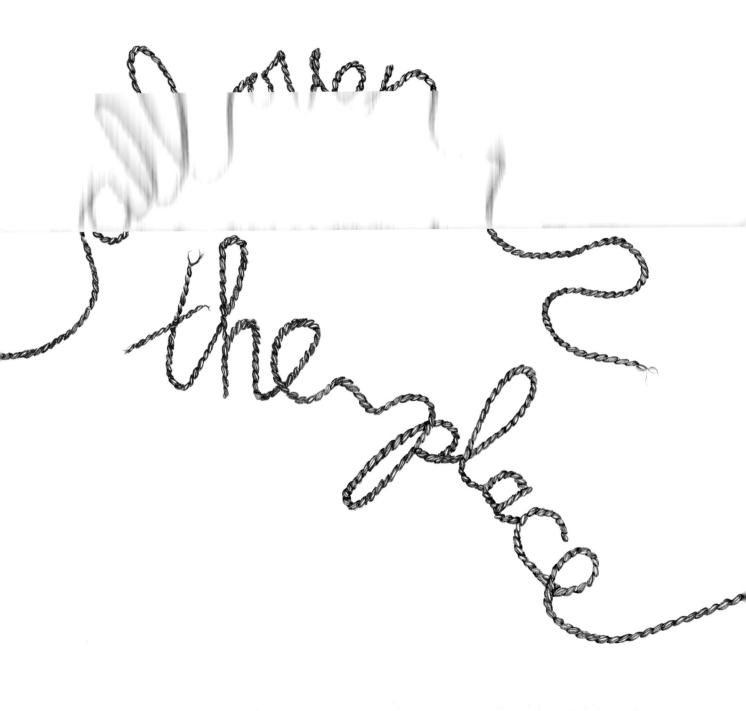

If you have any of these difficulties, it could be that you have dyslexia. About one in every ten people has it.

If you tell your teachers, there are lots of ways they can help you and lots of ways you can help yourself.

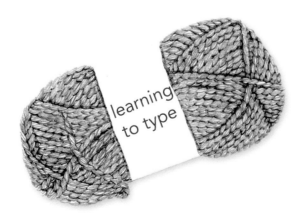

learning to type

reading and writing exercises

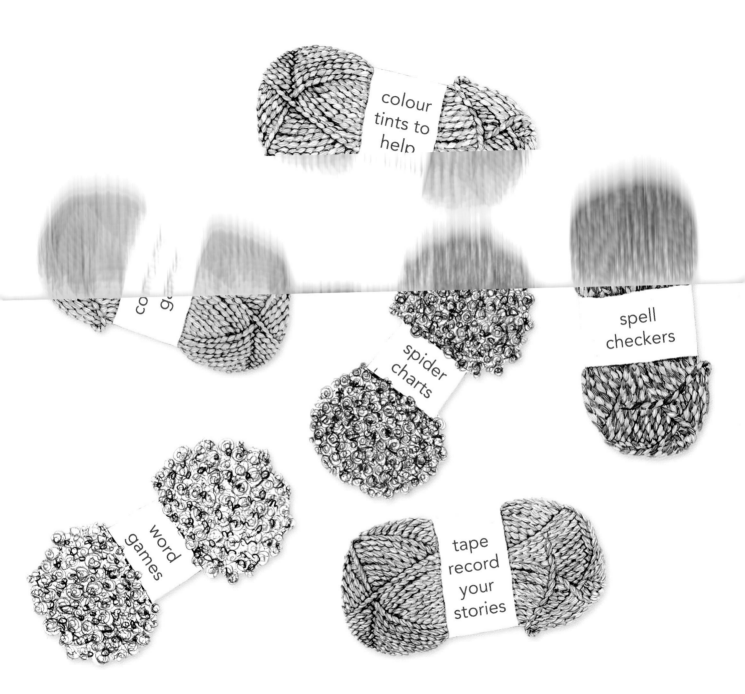

colour
tints to
help

co
g

spider
charts

spell
checkers

word
games

tape
record
your
stories

Then you can have…

fun with words and...

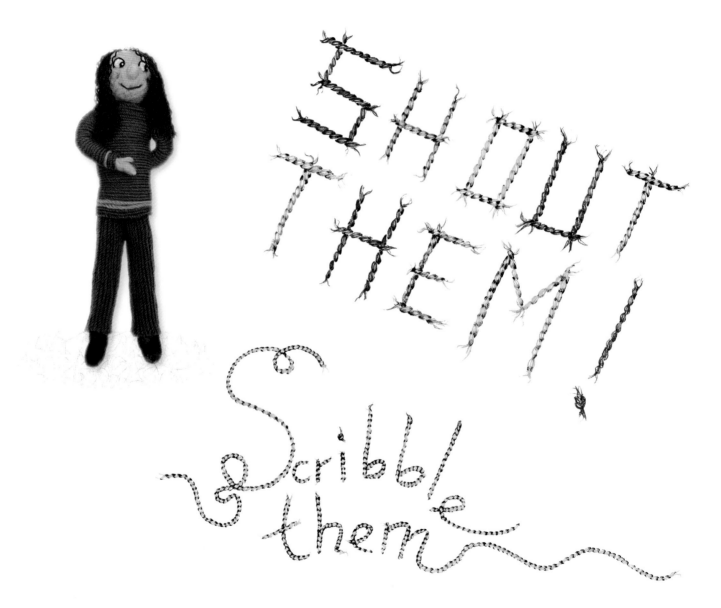

I SHOUT THEM!

Scribble them

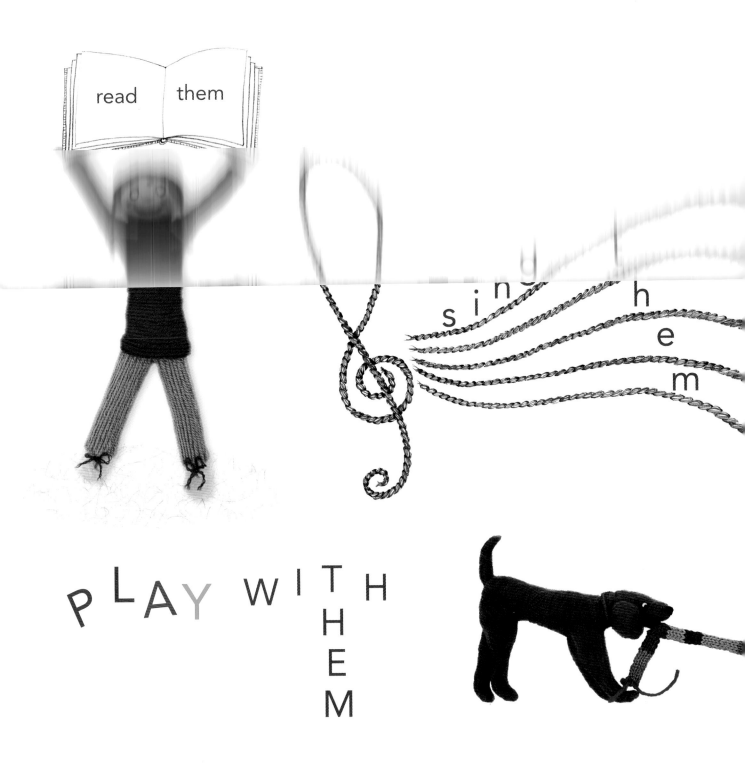

read them

sing them

PLAY WITH THEM

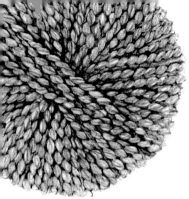

Everyone has talents and children with dyslexia are no different. They may be good at drama, maths, dancing, cookery, art or computing. They may be practical and creative.

There are many famous and talented people who have dyslexia, but you don't have to be famous to do well with it!

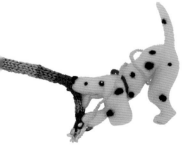

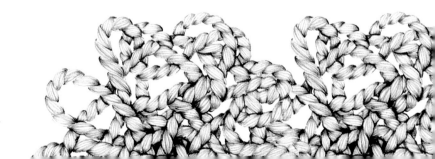

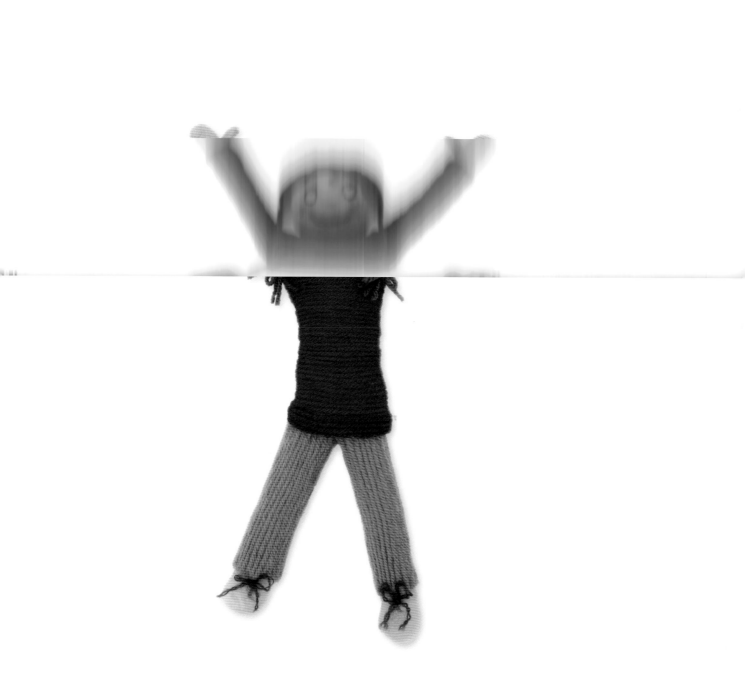

Ten Tips for Parents

All children learn through their senses – through what they see, what they hear and by acting upon materials that they handle. Children with dyslexia may experience difficulties with using the sense of sight to visually process information. They might also have problems remembering sounds and patterns that they hear such as the order of the alphabet letters or a sequence of instructions. Activities that involve touch and movement are *particularly* beneficial as not only are they more fun, but they also give the child's brain tactile and kinaesthetic as well as visual and auditory memories.

Make learning as active as possible:

1. Spread shaving foam, rice or couscous onto a tray. This can become your child's own 'writing tray'. They can use it to practise writing letter shapes, words or sentences.

2. For older children use whiteboards with whiteboard pens.

3. Give your child a washing up bottle or water pistol filled with water. Ask them to write letters or words on a hard surface outside such as a paved area or fence.

4. Let your child mix compost and water together. They can then use the 'mud' to write on hessian or old pillowcases with paintbrushes or sticks.

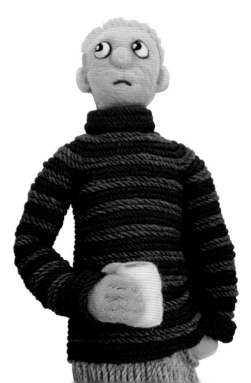

5. Make cakes and cookies with your child. Before you start, weigh the ingredients and put them into separate containers. Provide simple instructions for you and your child to read together e.g. 'Put in the eggs'.

8. Play memory games. Ask your child to put objects into a bag saying the name of the object as they put it in. They then pass the bag to another person and say, 'In the bag there is a…' As your child says the name of the object the other person removes it from the bag until there are no objects left.

9. Make sure everything has a place. Label boxes, drawers etc. with words and photos.

10. Break instructions into small chunks e.g. *'Get your school bag.'* Once the child has their school bag, give the next instruction.

Dyslexia is a difficulty with words and it is thought to be hereditary. If you are a parent and notice these difficulties in your child, then you, or someone else in your family may

If a child is helped to learn in the most appropriate way, dyslexia should not stop them reaching their full potential.

Sometimes dyslexia goes unnoticed because a child is seen to be 'coping' at school. It is just as important that these children's learning needs are understood.

Further information:
The British Dyslexia Association -
www.bdadyslexia.org

Dyslexia Action -
www.dyslexiaaction.org.uk

The Dyslexia Association of Ireland -
www.dyslexia.ie

Visual Thinking Specialist -
www.oliverwest.footnotes.com

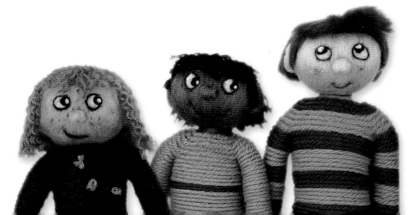

About the Author

When Pippa Sweeney's eldest daughter was found to have dyslexia at the age of twenty, she became passionate about raising dyslexia awareness. She was subsequently herself diagnosed with dyslexia, revealing the common hereditary link.

In 2011 Pippa completed an MA in Authorial Illustration at University College Falmouth in the UK, this book being researched and produced as part of her course.

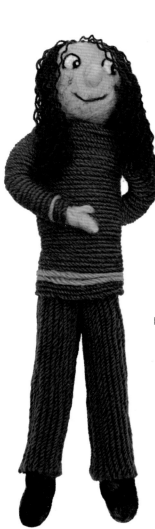

Having worked as an illustrator in London in the 1980's and spending a number of years in China, The Netherlands and New Zealand, Pippa now lives in Ireland with her husband, children, sheep and hens, where she writes and illustrates for children.

Dyslexia is a difficulty with words, and it is often misunderstood and sometimes unrecognised. If dyslexia remains undetected, it can affect a child's confidence and educational achievements.

This book's aim is to empower children with dyslexia to recognise and understand their own word difficulties and to teach their friends and family about it too!